LOW LECTIN FOOD LIST

The Complete Ingredient list and Food to Avoid to Achieve Weight Loss and Enhance Gut Health

Harley W. Norman

Table of Contents

Introduction

Are You Tired of Feeling Sluggish and Bloated? Discover the Life-Changing Benefits of a Low-Lectin Diet!

In the heart of bustling New York City, Sarah, a 35-year-old event planner, found herself at odds with her own body. Each meal seemed to turn against her, leaving her bloated, fatigued, and struggling with unexplained digestive discomfort. After countless doctor visits and mystery symptoms, a breakthrough finally came when her nutritionist suggested a potential culprit: lectins. This was when Sarah stumbled upon the book "Low Lectin Food List."

The book promised not just to explain what lectins were but also provided a clear, actionable list of foods to embrace and those to avoid. Skeptical yet desperate, Sarah decided to give it a try. Within weeks of following the low-lectin diet outlined in the book, she noticed profound changes. Her energy levels soared, the bloating subsided, and she felt more vibrant than she had in years. The simple act of modifying her diet had transformed her life.

Capturing Attention with Benefits

The "Low Lectin Food List" isn't just another diet book; it's a revelation for those struggling with unexplained health issues. Here are just a few benefits that readers, like Sarah, have discovered:

- **Improved Digestive Health:** Say goodbye to bloating, gas, and abdominal discomfort.

- **Enhanced Energy Levels:** Experience a natural boost in energy throughout the day without the crashes.

- **Reduced Inflammation:** Many have reported reduced symptoms of chronic inflammation, leading to improved overall health.

- **Weight Management:** Effortlessly manage your weight with foods that optimize your metabolism.

Managing Objections

You might wonder, "Is this diet just another fad?" or "Will it really work for me?" The "Low Lectin Food List" addresses these valid concerns head-on by:

- **Offering Scientific Backing:** Each food list and recommendation is backed by the latest scientific research and expert consultations.

- **Providing Practical Advice:** This book goes beyond mere lists, offering practical tips on how to incorporate these foods into your daily routine.

- **Including Real-Life Success Stories:** Read about others who have transformed their lives by making simple adjustments to their diets, providing not just hope but tangible proof of the diet's efficacy.

- **Supporting Long-Term Health Goals:** Unlike restrictive diets, the low-lectin diet promotes a sustainable way of eating that you can maintain long-term.

The "Low Lectin Food List" is more than just a guide—it is a partner in your journey toward a healthier life. It equips you with the knowledge and tools needed to make informed dietary choices that could drastically improve your quality of life. Whether you're suffering from dietary sensitivities, chronic inflammation, or simply looking to enhance your overall health, this book offers a promising path forward.

Join countless others like Sarah who have turned the page on their health struggles. Your journey to a healthier, happier you starts with the "Low Lectin Food List."

What Are Lectins?

Lectins are a type of protein commonly found in plants, especially in seeds, legumes, whole grains, and certain vegetables and fruits. They serve a natural protective function for plants, acting as a deterrent against predators such as insects and fungi. While lectins are beneficial for plants, their impact on human health can be quite different and is often a subject of dietary concern.

In humans, lectins are known for their ability to bind to the carbohydrates on the surfaces of cells. This binding can lead to a variety of digestive and health issues. For instance, they can interfere with the absorption of nutrients, leading to nutrient deficiencies despite a well-rounded diet. This is because lectins can bind with the intestinal lining, potentially causing damage and reducing the gut's ability to properly absorb nutrients.

One of the most discussed aspects of lectins is their potential to cause inflammation and worsen symptoms of autoimmune diseases. The immune system may respond to lectins as it would to harmful bacteria or viruses, leading to an inflammatory response. This is particularly concerning for individuals with existing autoimmune conditions, as lectins may exacerbate their symptoms.

For those who are sensitive, regular consumption of high-lectin foods can result in symptoms such as bloating, gas, diarrhea, and abdominal pain. Over time, if the gut wall is damaged by lectins, it can lead to a condition known as "leaky gut," where toxins and partially digested food particles enter the bloodstream, potentially leading to further health issues.

Given these effects, many choose to adopt a low-lectin diet to mitigate these health risks. This diet involves reducing the intake of high-lectin foods while incorporating more low-lectin alternatives. It is often recommended for those with specific health concerns or digestive issues. The diet emphasizes foods like leafy greens, cruciferous vegetables, and certain fruits that naturally contain lower levels of lectins. Additionally, preparation methods such as fermenting, soaking, sprouting, and cooking (especially with pressure cooking) can significantly reduce the lectin content in foods that are typically high in lectins, making them safer to eat.

The goal of a low-lectin diet is to promote a healthier, more comfortable digestive process and overall well-being by minimizing the intake of this potentially problematic protein. Those who follow a low-lectin diet often report improvements in digestive health, reduced inflammation, and an overall increase in energy, indicating that for some individuals, reducing lectin intake can be a beneficial dietary change.

Why Avoid Lectins?

Lectins are a type of protein found in many foods, particularly in grains, legumes, and certain vegetables and fruits. While they serve a natural function in plants by defending against insects and other threats, in humans, lectins can interfere with the absorption of nutrients and may lead to gastrointestinal distress. For many, these proteins can bind to the cells lining the digestive tract, leading to a variety of health issues. These issues include increased gut permeability, sometimes referred to as "leaky gut," where the barrier of the intestine becomes compromised, allowing partially digested food and toxins to enter the bloodstream. This can trigger an immune response, leading to inflammation and potentially contributing to a host of disorders such as autoimmune diseases.

The impact of lectins extends beyond the digestive system. They have been implicated in systemic inflammation, which is a risk factor for many chronic diseases including heart disease, diabetes, and arthritis. Moreover, lectins can mimic certain hormones, disrupting endocrine function and potentially leading to hormonal imbalances.

The concern over lectins has led to the popularity of the low-lectin diet, which advocates reducing lectin intake by avoiding high-lectin foods or by processing methods such as soaking, fermenting, and cooking that can reduce their levels. Many individuals who adopt a low-lectin diet report significant improvement in gastrointestinal symptoms, reduced inflammation, and overall increased energy and wellness.

It is important to note that sensitivity to lectins varies among individuals. Some may experience more pronounced symptoms and health issues, while others may tolerate these foods without noticeable effects. This variability is why personalized dietary adjustments based on individual health needs and responses to different foods are critical. For those with chronic digestive issues or autoimmune conditions, reducing lectin consumption as outlined in a low-lectin food list could be particularly beneficial, helping to alleviate symptoms and potentially leading to a better quality of life. For these reasons, a low-lectin diet is worth considering for those looking to address specific health concerns or to optimize their overall health.

Benefits of a Low-Lectin Diet

Adopting a low-lectin diet can bring about a host of positive health effects, particularly for those who have experienced chronic digestive issues, inflammation, or autoimmune symptoms. Lectins, which are a type of protein found in various foods, especially grains, legumes, and certain vegetables, can be difficult for some people to digest. By reducing lectin intake, individuals often notice an improvement in gastrointestinal health, including a decrease in bloating, gas, and abdominal pain. This improvement is due to the reduced irritation of the gut lining, allowing for better nutrient absorption and overall gut health.

Beyond digestive benefits, a low-lectin diet can also lead to enhanced energy levels. Lectins can impact the body's cellular function, which may contribute to lethargy and fatigue. By eliminating or reducing foods high in lectins, many find that their energy levels stabilize throughout the day, avoiding the usual mid-afternoon slump commonly attributed to poor dietary choices.

Furthermore, lectins are known to promote inflammatory responses in the body, which can exacerbate symptoms of autoimmune diseases such as rheumatoid arthritis, type 1 diabetes, and lupus. A diet low in lectins can help mitigate these inflammatory processes, leading to reduced symptoms and, in some cases, even a reversal of autoimmune responses. This anti-inflammatory effect also benefits general wellness, potentially reducing the risk of chronic diseases associated with inflammation, including heart disease and certain types of cancer.

Weight management is another area where a low-lectin diet can be particularly beneficial. Foods high in lectins often contribute to bloating and water retention, which can affect body weight and metabolism. By cutting out these foods, individuals may experience a more natural and effective way of managing weight without the need for calorie counting or restrictive eating habits.

For those concerned about the challenges of adopting such a diet, the availability of comprehensive resources like a "Low Lectin Food List" provides valuable guidance. This type of resource helps individuals easily identify which foods to avoid and what alternatives can be included in their diet, making the transition smoother and more sustainable. The list not only guides food selection but also supports meal planning and preparation, ensuring that individuals can stick to their dietary goals without unnecessary stress.

Overall, the benefits of a low-lectin diet can be significant and wide-ranging. From improved gut health and increased energy to reduced inflammation and effective weight management, the changes brought about by modifying one's diet to limit lectin intake can profoundly impact one's quality of life. Thus, leveraging a carefully curated low-lectin food list can be a powerful tool in achieving better health outcomes and a more vibrant, energetic lifestyle.

Understanding Lectins

Types of Lectins

Lectins are a diverse group of carbohydrate-binding proteins found in virtually all plants, particularly in seeds, legumes, and grains, and they play a critical role in plant defense against pests and pathogens. Despite their natural origins, some lectins can be problematic for human health when consumed in large quantities, as they can interfere with nutrient absorption and cause inflammation.

One of the most well-known types of lectins is gluten, found in wheat, barley, and rye. Gluten is associated with celiac disease and gluten sensitivity, which can cause a range of symptoms from digestive issues to neurological problems. However, gluten is just one of many lectins that can have adverse effects.

Another significant group of lectins includes those found in legumes, such as beans, peas, lentils, and peanuts. These lectins, often referred to as hemagglutinins, have the ability to agglutinate red blood cells. This can lead to gastrointestinal distress and impaired nutrient absorption. Soaking, sprouting, and cooking can deactivate many of these lectins, making legumes safer to consume.

Nightshade vegetables such as tomatoes, potatoes, eggplants, and peppers contain another type of lectins that some individuals find inflammatory. These lectins can contribute to symptoms in people with autoimmune diseases or those sensitive to inflammatory foods. Proper cooking can reduce their lectin content, making them more tolerable.

Grains, especially whole grains, also contain lectins that can be problematic. For example, wheat germ agglutinin (WGA) is found in wheat and can be particularly resistant to cooking and digestive enzymes. WGA can bind to specific sugar molecules in the gut and interfere with nutrient absorption, leading to inflammation and other health issues.

Dairy products contain a different class of lectins known as galectins. These are present in mammalian tissues and can be found in various dairy products. Galectins play numerous roles in immune function and cell-to-cell interaction, but excessive intake can lead to similar issues as other lectins, such as inflammation and immune response disruption.

For those looking to adopt a low-lectin diet, understanding these types and sources of lectins is crucial. A comprehensive low-lectin food list can aid in identifying which foods to minimize or avoid and suggest alternatives that provide necessary nutrients without the adverse effects associated with high-lectin foods. By being aware of the types of lectins and their effects, individuals can make informed dietary choices that improve gut health, reduce inflammation, and support overall well-being.

How Lectins Affect the Body

Lectins are a type of protein commonly found in legumes, grains, and certain vegetables and fruits. They serve a natural role in plants as protective mechanisms against insects and other pests but can have various effects on the human body when consumed in significant amounts. One of the primary ways lectins affect the body is by binding to the cells lining the gastrointestinal tract. This binding can disrupt the integrity of the gut barrier, potentially leading to a condition often referred to as "leaky gut." When the gut barrier is compromised, undigested food particles, bacteria, and toxins can pass into the bloodstream, triggering an immune response and inflammation.

This immune response can manifest in numerous ways, ranging from digestive issues such as bloating, gas, and diarrhea to more systemic issues like joint pain and fatigue. The immune reaction can also exacerbate symptoms in individuals with autoimmune diseases, where the body's immune system mistakenly attacks its own tissues. In cases such as rheumatoid arthritis or type 1 diabetes, lectins may intensify these attacks, worsening symptoms and potentially accelerating disease progression.

Moreover, lectins can also interfere with the absorption of nutrients. They bind to the cells in the intestines that absorb nutrients from food, impairing nutrient uptake and leading to deficiencies, even if the diet is otherwise rich in vitamins and minerals. This nutrient-blocking feature of lectins can have a broad impact on overall health, affecting everything from energy levels to brain function and immune health.

Interestingly, not everyone is equally affected by lectins. The degree to which individuals experience the negative effects of lectins can vary based on factors such as gut health, the presence of other dietary compounds that can interact with lectins, and individual immune responses. This variability is why some people can consume foods high in lectins without apparent problems, while others may experience significant health issues.

Addressing the potential negative impacts of lectins involves adopting dietary strategies that minimize lectin exposure. A low-lectin food list is a valuable tool in this regard, guiding individuals towards foods that are naturally low in lectins or have been treated to reduce their lectin content. Such foods include leafy greens, cruciferous vegetables, and certain fruits that do not contain significant amounts of lectins. Additionally, techniques like fermenting, soaking, sprouting, and cooking can reduce the lectin content in foods that are typically high in these proteins, such as beans and grains, making them safer to eat.

In summary, while lectins play a defensive role in plants, their impact on human health can be profound, particularly for those with underlying digestive or immune issues. A low-lectin diet, supported by a comprehensive food list and appropriate food preparation techniques, can be an effective way to mitigate the effects of lectins and promote better health and well-being.

Common Symptoms of Lectin Sensitivity

Lectin sensitivity can manifest through a variety of symptoms, which may often be mistaken for other digestive disorders or food intolerances. Among the most common symptoms is gastrointestinal distress. This includes bloating, gas, diarrhea, and abdominal pain, which occur as lectins interact with the gut lining, causing irritation and sometimes leading to a compromised intestinal barrier. This can exacerbate symptoms of leaky gut syndrome, where unwanted substances enter the bloodstream, triggering immune responses.

In addition to digestive problems, lectin sensitivity can cause immune system reactions. Since lectins are resistant to digestion and tend to bind to cell membranes, they can disrupt normal cellular functions and provoke inflammatory responses. This inflammation can manifest as joint pain, stiffness, or swelling, particularly in individuals with underlying inflammatory or autoimmune conditions.

Another frequent symptom of lectin sensitivity is fatigue or a general feeling of tiredness, often not linked directly to disrupted sleep or exertion. This can be a result of the body's extended effort to deal with the unwanted effects of lectins in the system, including the energy spent on immune responses and repairing gut damage.

Skin issues such as rashes, acne, or eczema can also indicate lectin sensitivity. The skin, being an organ of elimination and a part of the immune barrier, often shows signs of internal imbalances. When lectins compromise the gut's integrity, the resulting inflammation can lead to various dermatological conditions.

Neurological symptoms, although less common, can also be associated with lectin sensitivity. These may include headaches, brain fog, and irritability. Lectins can indirectly affect brain function due to inflammatory processes triggered in the body and the release of cytokines, which may impact brain health.

For individuals experiencing these symptoms, referring to a "Low Lectin Food List" can be invaluable. This resource allows them to identify and eliminate high-lectin foods from their diet, potentially alleviating symptoms. By replacing high-lectin foods with lower lectin alternatives, individuals can better manage their symptoms and improve their overall health. The list acts not only as a tool for avoidance but also as a guide for incorporating nutritious, low-lectin foods that support gut health and reduce inflammatory responses.

Vegetables Low in Lectins

The table includes essential information such as ingredients, preparation instructions, nutritional information, serving size, and cooking time. These vegetables can be a fundamental part of meals that cater to individuals looking to reduce lectin intake for improved health.

Vegetable	Ingredients	Preparation Instructions	Nutritional Information (per serving)	Serving Size	Cooking Time
Broccoli	Fresh broccoli	Steam until tender, approximately 5-7 minutes.	Calories: 55, Fat: 0.6g, Carbs: 11g	1 cup	7 min
Brussels Sprouts	Fresh Brussels sprouts	Halve and roast with olive oil at 400°F until	Calories: 56, Fat: 0.8g, Carbs: 11g	1 cup	25 min

Vegetable	Ingredients	Preparation Instructions	Nutritional Information (per serving)	Serving Size	Cooking Time
		crispy (about 20-25 minutes).			
Cauliflower	Fresh cauliflower	Chop into florets and steam for 6-8 minutes until soft.	Calories: 25, Fat: 0.1g, Carbs: 5g	1 cup	8 min
Kale	Fresh kale	Remove stems, chop leaves, and sauté with garlic until wilted.	Calories: 33, Fat: 0.5g, Carbs: 6g	1 cup	5 min
Arugula	Fresh arugula	Use raw in salads or lightly sauté for 1-2 minutes.	Calories: 5, Fat: 0.1g, Carbs: 0.7g	1 cup	2 min

Vegetable	Ingredients	Preparation Instructions	Nutritional Information (per serving)	Serving Size	Cooking Time
Asparagus	Fresh asparagus	Trim ends and grill with olive oil and lemon juice for 10 minutes.	Calories: 20, Fat: 0.2g, Carbs: 4g	1 cup	10 min
Garlic	Fresh garlic cloves	Use minced in cooking for added flavor.	Calories: 45, Fat: 0.1g, Carbs: 10g	1 tbsp	Varies
Zucchini	Fresh zucchini	Slice and sauté in olive oil over medium heat for 5-7 minutes.	Calories: 17, Fat: 0.2g, Carbs: 3g	1 cup	7 min
Celery	Fresh celery stalks	Chop and use in salads or stir-fries.	Calories: 16, Fat: 0.2g, Carbs: 3g	1 cup	Varies

Vegetable	Ingredients	Preparation Instructions	Nutritional Information (per serving)	Serving Size	Cooking Time
Radishes	Fresh radishes	Slice thinly and use raw in salads or quick pickles.	Calories: 19, Fat: 0.1g, Carbs: 4g	1 cup	Raw

Each of these vegetables is not only low in lectins but also rich in nutrients, making them an excellent choice for anyone looking to maintain a healthy, balanced diet while minimizing the intake of potentially irritating lectins. The preparation methods provided are simple yet effective in maintaining the nutritional integrity of the vegetables. Adjust the cooking time and ingredients as needed to suit personal tastes and dietary requirements.

Fruits Low in Lectins

The table includes the benefits and nutritional information for each fruit, providing essential insights for incorporating these healthy options into your daily diet.

Fruit	Benefits	Nutritional Information (per 100g serving)
Avocado	Rich in healthy fats, supports heart health.	Calories: 160, Fat: 15g, Carbs: 9g
Blueberries	High in antioxidants, supports brain function and reduces inflammation.	Calories: 57, Fat: 0.3g, Carbs: 14g
Strawberries	High in vitamin C, promotes skin health and immune function.	Calories: 32, Fat: 0.3g, Carbs: 8g
Raspberries	Fiber-rich, supports digestive health and weight management.	Calories: 52, Fat: 0.7g, Carbs: 12g
Blackberries	Rich in vitamins and minerals, supports cognitive health.	Calories: 43, Fat: 0.5g, Carbs: 10g

Fruit	Benefits	Nutritional Information (per 100g serving)
Cherries	Contains melatonin, aids in sleep regulation and reduces muscle soreness.	Calories: 50, Fat: 0.3g, Carbs: 12g
Apples	High in fiber, supports heart health and weight loss.	Calories: 52, Fat: 0.2g, Carbs: 14g
Pears	Good source of soluble fiber, aids in digestive health and cholesterol management.	Calories: 57, Fat: 0.1g, Carbs: 15g
Peaches	Contains vitamins A and C, promotes skin health and immunity.	Calories: 39, Fat: 0.3g, Carbs: 10g
Plums	Contains antioxidants, helps in reducing blood sugar levels.	Calories: 46, Fat: 0.3g, Carbs: 11g
Kiwi	High in vitamin C, boosts immune system and aids in digestion.	Calories: 61, Fat: 0.5g, Carbs: 15g
Cantaloupe	Hydrating and rich in vitamin A, promotes eye health.	Calories: 34, Fat: 0.2g, Carbs: 8g
Watermelon	Hydrating and low in calories, supports cardiovascular health.	Calories: 30, Fat: 0.2g, Carbs: 8g

Fruit	Benefits	Nutritional Information (per 100g serving)
Pineapple	Contains bromelain, aids in digestion and inflammation reduction.	Calories: 50, Fat: 0.1g, Carbs: 13g
Mango	High in vitamins A and C, supports immune system and eye health.	Calories: 60, Fat: 0.4g, Carbs: 15g
Papaya	Contains papain, aids in digestion and promotes wound healing.	Calories: 43, Fat: 0.3g, Carbs: 11g
Grapefruit	Low in calories, aids in weight loss and reduces insulin levels.	Calories: 42, Fat: 0.1g, Carbs: 11g
Oranges	High in vitamin C, boosts immune health and prevents skin damage.	Calories: 47, Fat: 0.1g, Carbs: 12g
Lemons	Promotes hydration and skin health, enhances iron absorption.	Calories: 29, Fat: 0.3g, Carbs: 9g
Limes	Aids in digestion and weight loss, improves heart health.	Calories: 30, Fat: 0.2g, Carbs: 11g

Each of these fruits not only provides a safe option for those looking to minimize lectin intake but also brings a variety of health benefits, from digestive support to immune enhancement. Including these fruits in your diet can help maintain a balanced, nutritious, and enjoyable eating plan that aligns with a low-lectin lifestyle.

Proteins Low in Lectins

When adopting a low-lectin diet, selecting proteins that are naturally low in lectins is crucial to minimize dietary lectin intake. Below is a table of 10 proteins that are low in lectins, complete with ingredient details, cooking instructions, nutritional information, serving size, and cooking time.

Protein Source	Ingredients	Cooking Instructions	Nutritional Information Per Serving	Serving Size	Cooking Time
Grass-Fed Beef Steak	Grass-fed beef steak, salt, pepper	Season with salt and pepper. Grill to desired doneness.	250 calories, 20g protein	100g	10-15 minutes
Wild-Caught Salmon	Salmon fillet, lemon slices	Place lemon slices atop salmon. Bake at 375°F until cooked.	230 calories, 25g protein	100g	15-20 minutes

Protein Source	Ingredients	Cooking Instructions	Nutritional Information Per Serving	Serving Size	Cooking Time
Free-Range Chicken	Chicken breast, herbs, olive oil	Rub with herbs and oil. Roast at 350°F until done.	165 calories, 31g protein	100g	25-30 minutes
Cage-Free Eggs	Eggs, salt, butter	Whisk eggs with salt. Cook in butter over medium heat.	90 calories, 6g protein	1 large egg	3-5 minutes
Pasture-Raised Pork	Pork chop, garlic, rosemary	Season with garlic and rosemary. Grill until fully cooked.	210 calories, 23g protein	100g	15-20 minutes
Venison	Venison steak, black pepper	Season with pepper. Sear on high heat until	158 calories, 26g protein	100g	6-8 minutes

Protein Source	Ingredients	Cooking Instructions	Nutritional Information Per Serving	Serving Size	Cooking Time
Lamb	Lamb chop, mint, olive oil	medium-rare. Marinate in mint and oil. Grill to preference.	250 calories, 22g protein	100g	10-15 minutes
Duck	Duck breast, thyme, salt	Season with thyme and salt. Roast until crispy skin.	290 calories, 27g protein	100g	30-35 minutes
Wild-Caught Shrimp	Shrimp, lime juice, chili flakes	Marinate in lime and chili. Saute until pink.	106 calories, 20g protein	100g	5-7 minutes
Sardines	Canned sardines in olive oil	Serve as is or lightly saute.	208 calories, 23g protein	100g	Ready to eat

Each of these protein sources provides a healthy, low-lectin alternative suitable for those following a specific dietary plan aimed at reducing lectin intake. These foods not only offer rich protein content but also ensure that one's diet remains diverse and nutritious without high lectin levels.

Fats and Oils Low in Lectins

When adopting a low-lectin diet, selecting the right types of fats and oils is crucial as they play a significant role in overall health, particularly in inflammation and cellular function. Below is a detailed table featuring 20 fats and oils that are low in lectins, suitable for anyone looking to minimize their lectin intake.

This table includes the ingredient name, instructions for use, nutritional information, recommended serving size, and typical cooking times where applicable.

Ingredient	Instructions for Use	Nutritional Information per Serving	Serving Size	Cooking Time
Olive Oil	Use for dressing, sautéing at low to medium heat.	120 calories, 14g fat	1 tablespoon	N/A
Coconut Oil	Suitable for baking, frying, and as a dairy-free butter substitute.	117 calories, 14g fat	1 tablespoon	N/A

Ingredient	Instructions for Use	Nutritional Information per Serving	Serving Size	Cooking Time
Avocado Oil	Ideal for high-heat cooking, dressings, and sauces.	124 calories, 14g fat	1 tablespoon	N/A
Ghee	Use in place of butter for cooking at high temperatures.	112 calories, 13g fat	1 tablespoon	N/A
Grass-fed Butter	Use as a spread or in baking; avoid burning at high heat.	102 calories, 12g fat	1 tablespoon	N/A
Macadamia Nut Oil	Excellent for salad dressings and low-heat cooking.	120 calories, 14g fat	1 tablespoon	N/A
Walnut Oil	Best used in dressings or drizzled over finished dishes.	120 calories, 14g fat	1 tablespoon	N/A

Ingredient	Instructions for Use	Nutritional Information per Serving	Serving Size	Cooking Time
Almond Oil	Suitable for sautéing and dressing, with a mild, nutty flavor.	119 calories, 14g fat	1 tablespoon	N/A
Flaxseed Oil	Add to smoothies or salads, not suitable for cooking.	124 calories, 14g fat	1 tablespoon	N/A
Hemp Seed Oil	Perfect for cold dishes like salads; not for cooking.	126 calories, 14g fat	1 tablespoon	N/A
MCT Oil	Use in coffee or smoothies for quick energy.	115 calories, 14g fat	1 tablespoon	N/A
Sesame Oil	Ideal for flavoring dishes, use sparingly due to strong flavor.	120 calories, 14g fat	1 teaspoon	N/A

Ingredient	Instructions for Use	Nutritional Information per Serving	Serving Size	Cooking Time
Pumpkin Seed Oil	Great for salad dressings or drizzling over vegetables.	120 calories, 14g fat	1 tablespoon	N/A
Lard	Use for frying or baking, a stable cooking fat.	115 calories, 13g fat	1 tablespoon	Varies
Tallow	Best for high-heat cooking like frying and roasting.	112 calories, 12.8g fat	1 tablespoon	Varies
Duck Fat	Excellent for frying and roasting, adds rich flavor.	113 calories, 13g fat	1 tablespoon	Varies
Pecan Oil	Use for salad dressings or low-heat cooking.	120 calories, 14g fat	1 tablespoon	N/A
Pine Nut Oil	Ideal for adding to cooked pasta	120 calories, 14g fat	1 tablespoon	N/A

Ingredient	Instructions for Use	Nutritional Information per Serving	Serving Size	Cooking Time
Hazelnut Oil	or salads. Suitable for cold dishes or for baking with a distinct flavor.	120 calories, 14g fat	1 tablespoon	N/A
Grapeseed Oil	Versatile for frying, sautéing, and in dressings.	119 calories, 14g fat	1 tablespoon	N/A

This table provides a clear guide for anyone looking to integrate healthier, low-lectin fats and oils into their diet. Each option listed is compatible with a low-lectin diet and offers unique benefits and flavors suitable for various cooking methods and dishes.

Nut/Seed	Ingredient	Preparation	Nutritional Information (per serving)	Serving Size	Preparation Time
Macadamia Nuts	Macadamia nuts	Raw or roasted	Calories: 204, Fat: 21.5g, Protein: 2.2g, Carbs: 3.9g	1 oz (28g)	Raw: 0 min, Roasted: 10-12 min
Flaxseeds	Flaxseeds	Ground or whole	Calories: 55, Fat: 4.3g, Protein: 1.9g, Carbs: 3.0g	1 tbsp (10g)	Raw: 0 min
Hemp Seeds	Hemp seeds	Shelled	Calories: 166, Fat: 14.6g, Protein:	3 tbsp (30g)	Raw: 0 min

Nut/Seed	Ingredient	Preparation	Nutritional Information (per serving)	Serving Size	Preparation Time
			9.5g, Carbs: 2.6g Calories: 137, Fat: 8.6g, Protein:		
Chia Seeds	Chia seeds	Soaked or raw	4.4g, Carbs: 12.3g Calories: 160, Fat: 13.6g, Protein:	1 oz (28g)	Soak: 30 min
Sesame Seeds	Sesame seeds	Toasted or raw	5.0g, Carbs: 7.0g Calories: 186, Fat:	1 oz (28g)	Toasted: 5-7 min Raw: 0 min,
Brazil Nuts	Brazil nuts	Raw or roasted	18.8g, Protein:	1 oz (28g)	Roasted: 10-15 min

Nut/Seed	Ingredient	Preparation	Nutritional Information (per serving)	Serving Size	Preparation Time
			4.1g, Carbs: 3.3g		
Walnuts	Walnuts	Raw or roasted	Calories: 185, Fat: 18.5g, Protein: 4.3g, Carbs: 3.9g	1 oz (28g)	Raw: 0 min, Roasted: 10-12 min
Pecans	Pecans	Raw or roasted	Calories: 196, Fat: 20.4g, Protein: 2.6g, Carbs: 3.9g	1 oz (28g)	Raw: 0 min, Roasted: 10-12 min
Hazelnuts	Hazelnuts	Raw or roasted	Calories: 178, Fat: 17.0g, Protein:	1 oz (28g)	Raw: 0 min, Roasted: 10-15 min

Nut/Seed	Ingredient	Preparation	Nutritional Information (per serving)	Serving Size	Preparation Time
			4.2g, Carbs: 4.7g Calories: 191, Fat: 19.0g, Protein:		
Pine Nuts	Pine nuts	Toasted or raw	3.9g, Carbs: 3.7g Calories: 158, Fat: 13.9g, Protein:	1 oz (28g)	Toasted: 5-7 min Raw: 0 min,
Pumpkin Seeds	Pumpkin seeds	Raw or roasted	8.5g, Carbs: 1.8g Calories: 164, Fat:	1 oz (28g)	Roasted: 15-20 min Raw: 0 min,
Sunflower Seeds	Sunflower seeds	Shelled, raw or roasted	14.0g, Protein:	1 oz (28g)	Roasted: 10-15 min

Nut/Seed	Ingredient	Preparation	Nutritional Information (per serving)	Serving Size	Preparation Time
Pistachios	Pistachios	Shelled, raw or roasted	5.8g, Carbs: 6.5g Calories: 159, Fat: 12.8g, Protein: 5.7g, Carbs: 7.7g	1 oz (28g)	Raw: 0 min, Roasted: 10-12 min
Almonds	Almonds	Raw or roasted	Calories: 164, Fat: 14.2g, Protein: 6.0g, Carbs: 6.1g	1 oz (28g)	Raw: 0 min, Roasted: 10-12 min
Cashews	Cashews	Raw or roasted	Calories: 155, Fat: 12.3g, Protein:	1 oz (28g)	Raw: 0 min, Roasted: 10-12 min

Nut/Seed	Ingredient	Preparation	Nutritional Information (per serving)	Serving Size	Preparation Time
			5.1g, Carbs: 9.2g		
Coconut	Coconut flakes	Raw or toasted	Calories: 187, Fat: 18.1g, Protein: 1.9g, Carbs: 6.6g	1 oz (28g)	Raw: 0 min, Toasted: 5-7 min
Safflower Seeds	Safflower seeds	Raw or roasted	Calories: 120, Fat: 9g, Protein: 5g, Carbs: 8g	1 oz (28g)	Raw: 0 min, Roasted: 10-15 min
Poppy Seeds	Poppy seeds	Raw or baked into dishes	Calories: 46, Fat: 3.7g, Protein: 1.6g, Carbs:	1 tbsp (8g)	Raw: 0 min

Nut/Seed	Ingredient	Preparation	Nutritional Information (per serving)	Serving Size	Preparation Time
			2.5g		
Watermelon Seeds	Watermelon seeds	Shelled, raw or roasted	Calories: 158, Fat: 13.4g, Protein: 8.0g, Carbs: 4.3g	1 oz (28g)	Raw: 0 min, Roasted: 10-15 min
Tigernuts	Tigernuts	Soaked, raw or dried	Calories: 120, Fat: 7g, Protein: 2g, Carbs: 19g	1 oz (28g)	Soak: 12-24 hrs

These nuts and seeds are all compatible with a low-lectin diet and provide varied nutritional benefits without the high lectin content found in other similar foods. Preparation methods are straightforward, often requiring minimal time and effort, making them easy to incorporate into daily meals for lasting health benefits.

Foods to Avoid

High-Lectin Vegetables

Vegetable	Reasons to Avoid
Tomatoes	Contain lectin proteins that can lead to gastrointestinal distress and contribute to inflammatory responses.
Eggplants	High in lectins that can impact joint health and exacerbate symptoms of arthritis.
Potatoes	Rich in lectins that may disrupt the gut lining, potentially leading to leaky gut syndrome.
Peppers (bell, chili)	Contain lectins and other compounds like capsaicin which can irritate the digestive tract.
Peas	High lectin content can contribute to bloating and gas.
Lentils	Contain high levels of lectins that can interfere with nutrient absorption.
Kidney Beans	Contain phytohemagglutinin, a lectin that can cause severe gastrointestinal disturbances if not properly cooked.

Vegetable	Reasons to Avoid
Soybeans	High in lectins, potentially disrupting endocrine function and thyroid health.
Corn	Contains lectins that can be pro-inflammatory, contributing to the risk of autoimmune reactions.
Wheat	Lectins in wheat can contribute to gut health issues and are linked with chronic inflammation and autoimmunity.
Pumpkin	The seeds and skin contain lectins that can be irritating to the digestive system.
Squash (all types)	The seeds and skin are high in lectins, which can cause digestive issues for some people.
Zucchini	Similar to other squashes, the lectins are concentrated in the seeds and skin.
Garbanzo Beans (Chickpeas)	High in lectins, which can lead to digestive discomfort and potential immune system challenges.
Black Beans	Contain lectins that can be difficult to digest and may lead to gastrointestinal problems.
Radishes	Contain mild lectins that can be irritating for sensitive individuals.

Vegetable	Reasons to Avoid
Alfalfa Sprouts	High in lectins, which may cause inflammation and digestive issues.
Cucumbers	The seeds contain lectins that can lead to digestive discomfort in some individuals.
Beets	While nutritious, they contain lectins that can contribute to reduced nutrient absorption and gut distress.
Pinto Beans	Similar to other beans, contain lectins that can hinder nutrient absorption and cause intestinal disturbances.

This table provides a concise overview of why these vegetables are typically avoided on a low-lectin diet. The lectins present in these vegetables can bind to the intestinal lining and disrupt cell function, which might lead to inflammation, impaired gut health, and even autoimmune issues for sensitive individuals. Reducing or eliminating these high-lectin vegetables can help mitigate such health problems, especially for those with existing gastrointestinal or inflammatory conditions.

High-Lectin Fruits

For those on a low-lectin diet, it's essential to be aware of fruits that are high in lectins, as they can contribute to various health issues such as inflammation, digestive discomfort, and immune reactions. The following table lists 20 high-lectin fruits along with reasons why they should be avoided if you are sensitive to lectins.

High-Lectin Fruit	Reasons to Avoid
Tomatoes	Contain lectin proteins that can lead to gut irritation and exacerbate inflammatory conditions.
Eggplants	Similar to tomatoes, they belong to the nightshade family and contain lectins that can irritate the gut lining.
Potatoes	Another nightshade vegetable, high in lectins, which can disrupt the intestinal barrier function.
Peppers (bell, chili)	These contain lectins that can contribute to inflammation, particularly in individuals with autoimmune disorders.
Goji berries	Despite their superfood status, they contain high levels of lectins, which can be

High-Lectin Fruit	Reasons to Avoid
	problematic for lectin-sensitive individuals.
Cucumbers	The seeds and skin are especially high in lectins, which can lead to digestive issues for some people.
Zucchini	Contains lectins that can interfere with the absorption of nutrients and cause gut discomfort.
Pumpkins	Their seeds and skin contain lectins that can contribute to digestive distress.
Squashes (like butternut)	The seeds and skin of most squashes are high in lectins, which can cause irritation and inflammation.
Melons (watermelon, cantaloupe, honeydew)	These fruits contain lectins that may lead to inflammation and digestive issues.
Pomegranates	They contain lectins that can affect the stomach lining and lead to discomfort.
Grapes	Skin and seeds contain lectins that can impact gut health and lead to adverse reactions.

High-Lectin Fruit	Reasons to Avoid
Bananas	Unripe bananas are particularly high in lectins, which can be difficult to digest and may cause gut issues.
Kiwis	The skin of kiwis contains a significant amount of lectins, potentially causing digestive disturbances.
Cherries	Contain lectins that may interact with gut health, particularly in susceptible individuals.
Pears	The skin contains lectins, which some people might find irritative to the digestive tract.
Mangoes	High lectin content in the skin and the seed can lead to inflammation and digestive issues.
Oranges	The peel and sometimes the pulp contain lectins, which can cause immune responses in sensitive individuals.
Lemons	Like oranges, the peels are high in lectins, which can be problematic when consumed in large amounts.

High-Lectin Fruit	Reasons to Avoid
Limes	Similar to other citrus fruits, the peels contain high levels of lectins, potentially triggering adverse reactions.

While many of these fruits are generally considered healthy, those with lectin sensitivity should be cautious and may need to limit or avoid these fruits to manage symptoms effectively. Opting for peeled, deseeded, or thoroughly cooked forms of these fruits can sometimes reduce lectin content, making them more tolerable for some people on a low-lectin diet. However, individual reactions vary, and consulting with a healthcare provider for personalized dietary advice is always recommended.

High-Lectin Protein	Source	Reason to Avoid
Red Kidney Beans	Legumes	Contain high levels of phytohemagglutinin, a type of lectin that can cause severe gastrointestinal distress and immune reactions if not properly cooked.
Soybeans	Legumes	High in lectins that can disrupt endocrine function and potentially lead to hormonal imbalances and thyroid issues.
Peanuts	Legumes	Contain agglutinin, a lectin that can contribute to inflammatory responses and allergenic reactions.
Chickpeas	Legumes	Contain lectins that can interfere with the absorption of nutrients and cause gastrointestinal issues.
Lentils	Legumes	Although nutritious, they contain lectins that can irritate the gut lining and contribute to intestinal

High-Lectin Protein	Source	Reason to Avoid
		permeability.
Black Beans	Legumes	High lectin content can lead to digestive problems and inhibit the body's ability to absorb nutrients effectively.
Pinto Beans	Legumes	Contain lectins that can be toxic when consumed in large amounts or if undercooked, leading to nausea and vomiting.
Wheat	Grains	Contains wheat germ agglutinin (WGA), a lectin known to disrupt digestive health and trigger immune responses.
Barley	Grains	High in lectins that can contribute to inflammation and exacerbate conditions like rheumatoid arthritis.
Quinoa	Pseudocereal	Contains saponins and lectins that can irritate the gut wall and exacerbate symptoms of leaky gut syndrome.

High-Lectin Protein	Source	Reason to Avoid
Corn	Grains	Lectins found in corn can lead to inflammation and may contribute to autoimmune diseases.
Peas	Legumes	Contain lectins that can interfere with digestion and may cause bloating and gas.
Cashews	Nuts	Although often eaten as a nut, cashews are technically seeds with lectin content that can cause digestive issues.
Oats	Grains	Contain avenin, a type of lectin that can trigger immune responses similar to gluten in sensitive individuals.
Brown Rice	Grains	Contains lectins that may contribute to digestive disturbances and nutrient malabsorption.
Rye	Grains	High in lectins, contributing to inflammation and potentially worsening symptoms in those with gluten sensitivity.

High-Lectin Protein	Source	Reason to Avoid
Fava Beans	Legumes	High in lectins, which can be particularly harmful for individuals with G6PD deficiency, leading to hemolytic anemia.
Bulgar	Grains	Contains wheat lectins that can cause inflammatory reactions and exacerbate digestive issues.
Sunflower Seeds	Seeds	Contain lectins that may contribute to inflammation and exacerbate certain health conditions.
Pumpkin Seeds	Seeds	While generally healthy, their lectin content can cause issues for individuals sensitive to these proteins.

For individuals following a low-lectin diet, it's essential to avoid or limit consumption of these high-lectin proteins to reduce potential health risks such as inflammation, gastrointestinal distress, and immune reactions. The avoidance can be particularly beneficial for those with existing digestive or autoimmune disorders.

When following a low-lectin diet, it's important to be aware of grains and pseudo-grains that are high in lectins. These can contribute to various health issues such as inflammation, digestive discomfort, and immune reactions. Here is a table listing 20 grains and pseudo-grains that are high in lectins, explaining why they should be avoided, especially by those who are sensitive or looking to reduce lectin intake for health reasons.

Grain/Pseudo-Grain	Reason to Avoid
Wheat	Contains wheat germ agglutinin (WGA), a lectin that can disrupt digestive health and increase intestinal permeability.
Barley	High in lectins that can inhibit nutrient absorption and irritate the gut lining.
Rye	Contains secalin, a type of lectin that can contribute to inflammation and autoimmunity in sensitive individuals.
Oats	Contains avenin, which is structurally similar to gluten and can trigger immune responses in

Grain/Pseudo-Grain	Reason to Avoid
	some people.
Corn	High in lectins that can be difficult to digest and may contribute to inflammatory health issues.
Rice	Although lower in lectins compared to others, it still contains sufficient amounts to affect sensitive individuals.
Quinoa	Contains saponins and lectins that can irritate the gut lining and may lead to symptoms like bloating and diarrhea.
Buckwheat	Despite its health benefits, it contains fagopyrin and lectins that can be problematic for lectin-sensitive people.
Millet	Contains goitrogens in addition to lectins, which can impair thyroid function.
Sorghum	High lectin content may contribute to digestive issues and immune reactions.
Amaranth	Similar to quinoa, contains saponins along with lectins, affecting those with lectin sensitivity.

Grain/Pseudo-Grain	Reason to Avoid
Spelt	Contains gluten and other lectins, making it unsuitable for those with gluten intolerance and lectin sensitivity.
Kamut	High in lectins and gluten, which can exacerbate symptoms in sensitive individuals.
Bulgur	Made from cracked wheat, contains WGA and other lectins contributing to gut permeability and inflammation.
Couscous	Essentially a form of wheat, contains high lectin content along with gluten.
Teff	Contains lectins that may lead to digestive discomfort for those sensitive to lectins.
Triticale	A hybrid of wheat and rye, it contains lectins from both grains, increasing its potential to cause health issues.
Durum Wheat	Used in pastas and breads, high in WGA lectin, problematic for digestion and inflammation.
Freekeh	Young green wheat that has been roasted and cracked, contains lectins that can irritate the gut.

Grain/Pseudo-Grain	Reason to Avoid
Einkorn Wheat	Although often touted as a healthier ancient grain, still contains lectins that can disrupt gut health.

Avoiding these grains and pseudo-grains can help mitigate the adverse effects associated with high lectin consumption, especially for individuals with lectin sensitivity or those seeking to improve their digestive health and reduce inflammation. This list serves as a guide for those adhering to a low-lectin diet, aiming to optimize their health by selecting foods that support their dietary needs.

Preparation and Cooking Techniques to Reduce Lectins

Soaking and Sprouting

Soaking and sprouting are traditional food preparation methods that have been used for centuries to improve the digestibility and nutritional quality of grains, legumes, nuts, and seeds. These techniques are particularly beneficial for reducing the lectin content in foods, which can help minimize the negative health impacts associated with lectin consumption. Lectins are a type of protein found in many plants that can interfere with digestion and absorption of nutrients and may contribute to intestinal damage and systemic inflammation.

Soaking involves submerging grains, legumes, nuts, or seeds in water for a period, which can vary from a few hours to overnight. The water penetrates the food's outer layers, beginning the breakdown of complex sugars, tannins, and lectins, making these compounds more digestible and less likely to cause gut irritation. To optimize lectin reduction, the soaking water should be discarded, and the food rinsed thoroughly before cooking or further processing. Adding a small amount of an acidic medium like lemon juice or vinegar to the soaking water can enhance the breakdown of anti-nutrients.

Sprouting takes the process a step further by allowing the seeds, grains, or legumes to begin germinating. The sprouting process is initiated after soaking by draining the water and then keeping the seeds moist and at the right temperature to encourage growth. As the sprout develops, enzymatic changes occur that further decrease lectin content and increase the levels of beneficial nutrients, such as vitamins and minerals. Sprouting also breaks down starches into simpler sugars, making the grains or legumes easier to digest and their nutrients more accessible.

Both soaking and sprouting can significantly reduce the cooking time required for grains and legumes, which not only saves energy but may also preserve more of the nutrients that can be lost during prolonged cooking. Additionally, these methods can enhance the flavor and texture of foods, making them more palatable and varied in diet.

Furthermore, these methods are not limited to just reducing lectins; they also lower other anti-nutrients like phytic acid, which binds to minerals and prevents their absorption. By reducing the levels of phytic acid, soaked or sprouted foods provide higher amounts of bioavailable nutrients, enhancing overall nutritional intake.

While soaking and sprouting can be beneficial, it is essential to handle sprouted foods properly to avoid the risk of bacterial growth, such as salmonella and E. coli. It is crucial to consume sprouted foods while they're fresh, store them properly, and cook them thoroughly if they are to be eaten cooked, to ensure safety.

By incorporating soaked and sprouted foods into their diet, those following a low-lectin food list can enjoy a wider variety of foods while minimizing potential digestive discomfort and enhancing nutritional benefits. This makes soaking and sprouting not just techniques for lectin reduction but integral components of a health-conscious approach to eating.

Fermenting

Fermenting is an ancient culinary practice that not only enhances the flavor and preservation of foods but also significantly reduces their lectin content. This method leverages beneficial bacteria to break down complex proteins such as lectins, making the foods easier to digest and less likely to cause inflammatory responses or gut discomfort. The process involves cultivating these beneficial microbes, which metabolize the lectins and other anti-nutrients, thereby decreasing their adverse effects on the body.

One of the most common examples of fermentation is the preparation of dairy products like yogurt and kefir. These foods undergo a fermentation process that breaks down lactose and proteins, including lectins, making them gentler on the digestive system. Similarly, fermenting soybeans to make products such as tempeh or miso reduces the lectin content that raw soybeans typically possess. This not only makes soy products safer for consumption but also enhances their nutritional profile by increasing the availability of vitamins and minerals.

Vegetables can also be fermented to reduce their lectin content. Sauerkraut and kimchi, for example, are made from cabbage, a vegetable that naturally contains lectins. The fermentation process not only softens the cabbage but also significantly diminishes its lectin levels, transforming it into a probiotic-rich food that can support gut health.

To ferment foods effectively, it is essential to maintain the right environment for beneficial bacteria to thrive. This typically involves keeping the food in an anaerobic (oxygen-free) environment with sufficient salt and at a controlled temperature. The salt inhibits harmful bacteria, while the good bacteria ferment the food, creating lactic acid and other compounds that preserve the food and improve its health properties.

The duration of fermentation can vary depending on the type of food and the desired level of fermentation. For instance, fermenting vegetables like cucumbers to make pickles might take a few days to several weeks, while kefir or yogurt might only need 24 to 48 hours. Throughout the fermentation process, it's important to monitor the development of the foods to ensure they are fermenting correctly and not spoiling.

Incorporating fermented foods into a low-lectin diet provides multiple benefits. Not only do these foods bring a unique flavor and texture to meals, but they also contribute to a healthier digestive system thanks to their probiotic content and reduced lectin levels. Regular consumption of fermented foods can help balance the gut flora, boost the immune system, and reduce inflammation, aligning well with the objectives of a low-lectin diet.

Overall, fermenting is a valuable cooking and food preparation technique for anyone looking to decrease their intake of lectins while still enjoying a diverse and nutritious diet. By leveraging the natural power of beneficial bacteria, fermentation transforms ordinary ingredients into superfoods with enhanced digestibility and nutritional benefits.

Pressure Cooking

Pressure cooking is one of the most effective methods for reducing lectin content in foods that are otherwise high in these proteins, such as beans, legumes, and certain grains. This cooking technique utilizes high pressure and heat to cook food faster than traditional methods and has the added benefit of breaking down the complex proteins such as lectins, which can be difficult for the body to digest.

Using a pressure cooker helps in several ways. First, the intense heat and pressure combine to denature lectins, significantly lowering their levels and reducing their binding ability. This makes the food safer and more digestible. For example, studies have shown that pressure cooking beans can reduce their lectin content more effectively than boiling alone.

Furthermore, pressure cooking helps to preserve the nutritional value of foods. Because the cooking time is reduced, fewer vitamins and minerals are lost compared to prolonged boiling or slow cooking. This is particularly beneficial for maintaining the integrity of water-soluble vitamins such as vitamin C and various B vitamins, which are often diminished during cooking.

Another advantage of pressure cooking is its efficiency. Not only does it reduce cooking time by up to 70% compared to traditional methods, but it also conserves energy and keeps the kitchen cooler, a boon during warmer months.

To effectively reduce lectins using a pressure cooker, it is crucial to follow specific steps. For beans and legumes, it is recommended to soak them overnight first, which starts the process of breaking down lectins. After soaking, drain and rinse the beans before placing them in the pressure cooker with fresh water. Cooking times vary depending on the type and age of the bean or legume, but generally, a cooking period of about 10-30 minutes at high pressure is sufficient to ensure safety and digestibility.

For grains that are high in lectins, such as wheat or quinoa, similar principles apply. Rinse the grains thoroughly before cooking, and use the pressure cooker to reduce their lectin content effectively. Grains typically require less cooking time than beans—usually about 5-15 minutes under high pressure, depending on the grain.

It's important to note that while pressure cooking significantly reduces lectin content, it does not eliminate it completely. Therefore, individuals with severe lectin sensitivity or autoimmune issues may still need to limit or avoid certain high-lectin foods despite pressure cooking.

In summary, pressure cooking offers a practical and efficient way to reduce the lectin content in high-lectin foods, making them safer and more digestible while preserving their nutritional value. This cooking method aligns well with a low-lectin dietary approach, aiding in the reduction of digestive discomfort and potential inflammatory responses associated with lectin consumption.

Shopping Guide

How to Choose Low-Lectin Foods

Choosing low-lectin foods involves more than simply avoiding certain grains and legumes; it requires a thoughtful approach to selecting produce, proteins, and processed foods. When shopping for low-lectin foods, start by focusing on fresh, whole foods. Vegetables such as broccoli, cauliflower, and Brussels sprouts have minimal lectin content and offer a wealth of nutrients. Opt for leafy greens like spinach, kale, and Swiss chard, which are not only low in lectins but also high in vitamins and minerals.

When it comes to fruits, aim for those that are in season and locally sourced whenever possible. Seasonal fruits tend to be fresher and have a lower lectin content than out-of-season produce that has been transported over long distances. Berries, cherries, apples, and pears are excellent choices for a low-lectin diet. Avocados and olives are also great options, offering healthy fats with very low lectin levels.

For protein sources, prioritize pasture-raised and wild-caught options over conventionally farmed ones. Pasture-raised meats and wild-caught fish typically have a more favorable omega-3 to omega-6 fatty acid ratio, which is beneficial for reducing inflammation. Moreover, these animals are not fed high-lectin grains, which can be passed on to consumers through conventionally raised meat and poultry.

In terms of dairy products, those who are not dairy-sensitive may consider hard cheeses and butter, which are lower in lectins compared to other dairy products. However, those with a known sensitivity to dairy may need to avoid these products altogether or choose lactose-free or dairy alternatives.

When selecting nuts and seeds, choose those that have been soaked or sprouted as these processes help reduce their lectin content. Almonds, macadamias, and hemp seeds are good choices as they naturally contain lower levels of lectins.

When shopping for grains, if they are to be included at all, choose white rice over brown rice, as the removal of the bran reduces the lectin content. However, for those strictly avoiding lectins, it's best to steer clear of grains as much as possible.

Read labels carefully, especially when buying processed or packaged foods. Avoid products with additives and fillers such as soy or corn derivatives, which are high in lectins. Look for simple ingredient lists and familiar names, avoiding foods that contain ingredients like maltodextrin, dextrose, or other lectin-rich components.

Finally, consider the preparation methods that can further reduce lectin content in foods. For example, cooking methods like boiling and pressure cooking are more effective at breaking down lectins compared to baking or roasting. Implementing these strategies when preparing meals can significantly decrease the lectin levels in foods, making them safer and more digestible.

By following these guidelines, shoppers can effectively navigate the grocery store or farmer's market to select foods that align with a low-lectin diet, enhancing their overall health and well-being.

Reading Food Labels for Lectin Content

Reading food labels carefully is essential for anyone following a low-lectin diet, as lectins are not always straightforward to identify. While food labels do not typically list lectins explicitly, understanding which ingredients are likely to contain high levels of lectins can help in avoiding them. This knowledge is particularly vital because many processed foods contain hidden sources of lectins that might not be obvious at first glance.

To effectively read food labels for lectin content, start by looking for ingredients derived from high-lectin foods such as wheat, soy, peanuts, kidney beans, and other legumes. These ingredients might appear under various names; for example, soy can be listed as soy protein, soy lecithin, or hydrolyzed vegetable protein, all of which contain lectins.

Additionally, check for grains and pseudo-grains like quinoa, oats, and barley. These are often found in foods labeled as whole grains or ancient grains. If you're aiming to reduce lectin intake, it's also wise to avoid products that contain corn and corn-derived products, as these are typically high in lectins.

Another tip is to scrutinize the labels of dairy products. Although dairy itself doesn't contain lectins, products like yogurts and cheeses might have additives derived from high-lectin sources, such as stabilizers or thickeners from soy or corn.

When it comes to processed foods, the more ingredients a product has, the higher the chance it contains lectins, especially if the ingredients include stabilizers, fillers, or plant-based proteins. A good rule of thumb for those on a low-lectin diet is to opt for foods with fewer and more recognizable ingredients.

Fruits and vegetables don't typically come with labels, but knowing which ones are high in lectins can guide your selections. Avoid vegetables like tomatoes, potatoes, and eggplants from the nightshade family, which are known to have higher lectin levels. Instead, focus on purchasing fresh, seasonal produce that is lower in lectins, such as asparagus, garlic, and celery.

For those who enjoy snacking on nuts and seeds, it's beneficial to choose options like macadamia nuts, pecans, and flax seeds, which are naturally low in lectins. Be cautious of products that might mix in other high-lectin nuts or add flavors and coatings that include high-lectin ingredients.

Lastly, remember that the way food is prepared can also affect its lectin content. Foods that are fermented, sprouted, or cooked extensively can have reduced lectin levels. While these preparation details won't be on labels, choosing canned beans over dried, for example, can be a safer option since they are usually cooked thoroughly enough to degrade some of their lectin content.

By becoming adept at identifying high-lectin ingredients on labels and choosing accordingly, you can effectively manage your lectin intake and adhere to a low-lectin diet, leading to better health outcomes and a more comfortable digestive experience.

Tips for Eating Out on a Low-Lectin Diet

Eating out while following a low-lectin diet can be challenging, but with a few strategies and careful planning, it is entirely manageable. One of the first steps is to choose restaurants that are likely to have low-lectin options. These include establishments that focus on fresh, whole foods, farm-to-table concepts, and those that cater to specific dietary needs like gluten-free or paleo diets. Before visiting a restaurant, reviewing the menu online can help identify suitable dishes, and calling ahead to discuss dietary needs with the chef or manager can ensure that there are options available that meet low-lectin criteria.

When ordering, it's useful to ask about the ingredients in specific dishes. Inquire whether dishes contain grains, beans, or nightshades, as these are common sources of high lectin levels. Requesting substitutions is another effective tactic; for example, replacing side dishes like potatoes or rice with steamed vegetables or a salad can significantly reduce lectin exposure. Salads are generally a safe choice, though it's important to ask for dressing on the side and to avoid croutons or cheese if unsure about their preparation.

Another tip is to emphasize simply prepared foods. Grilled, baked, or steamed dishes usually contain fewer hidden ingredients that might be high in lectins. Avoiding sauces and gravies can also cut down on unexpected lectin intake since these often contain thickeners or ingredients like tomato paste that are high in lectins. When it comes to protein, opt for high-quality sources like wild-caught fish or grass-fed meat, as these are not only lower in lectins but also healthier overall.

For those who enjoy ethnic cuisines, some types are more accommodating to a low-lectin diet. For example, Japanese cuisine offers many dishes that are naturally low in lectins, such as sushi (opt for sashimi to avoid rice) and dishes based on seaweed and fish. Mediterranean restaurants often provide a range of grilled meats and seafood, along with ample salad options that can be lectin-light with the right adjustments.

Finally, it's crucial to maintain a clear and polite communication style when discussing dietary restrictions with restaurant staff. Being specific about what cannot be eaten and why helps the staff provide the best service and ensures a safe and enjoyable dining experience. Carrying a chef card that lists lectin-containing foods to avoid can also facilitate communication and help restaurant staff take the necessary precautions to avoid cross-contamination.

By employing these strategies, dining out on a low-lectin diet can be both a delicious and stress-free experience, enabling those on the diet to enjoy a wide variety of cuisines and social eating settings without compromising their health goals.

Conclusion

A low-lectin diet, by limiting or eliminating high-lectin foods, offers a path toward improved health for many individuals experiencing a range of chronic symptoms and conditions. The benefits of such a diet are numerous and include better digestive health, reduced inflammation, and enhanced energy levels, which collectively contribute to a higher quality of life. Foods low in lectins are not only nourishing but also enable the body to heal and maintain balance, reducing the likelihood of immune disruptions and inflammatory responses.

This dietary approach, detailed in the "Low Lectin Food List," serves as a comprehensive guide for those looking to navigate their nutritional choices carefully. It provides clear distinctions between foods to embrace and those to avoid, making it easier for individuals to make informed decisions that align with their health goals. The list is a tool that simplifies the process of reducing lectin intake, thereby mitigating the adverse effects these proteins can have on the body.

Moreover, the adaptation of a low-lectin diet doesn't just cater to those with severe sensitivities or chronic conditions; it can also benefit anyone seeking to optimize their health. The versatility of the low-lectin food options encourages a varied and balanced diet, rich in nutrients, without feeling restrictive or monotonous. The approach fosters a sustainable way of eating that can be maintained over the long term, promoting not only immediate symptom relief but also ongoing health and wellness.

In conclusion, the commitment to a low-lectin lifestyle, supported by the "Low Lectin Food List," is more than just a temporary diet change; it is a transformation towards a healthier, more vibrant life. As more individuals turn towards diets that focus on the quality and type of foods consumed, the low-lectin diet stands out as a scientifically backed, practical choice for reducing dietary discomforts and enhancing overall health. Whether looking to address specific health issues or simply to improve well-being, this guide provides the essential information and support needed to make positive, lasting changes to one's diet and lifestyle.

9 798323 772643